Torticollis

A Complete Care Guide

Causes, Symptoms, and Treatment all covered!

By: Frederick Earlstein

Foreword

The structure of the human neck allows for a wide range of motion we take for granted in our daily lives. When we drop our chin toward our chests we don't consciously think, "flexion," any more than we deliberately measure the possible range of rotation out of neutral to a normal 45-70 degrees. But then something goes wrong.

Sometimes it's just a "crick" — pain or stiffness — often from sleeping in a strange position. Once the muscles get "warmed up," maybe even with the application of actual heat, the spasm loosens up and we're able to use our necks normally again.

But if the neck twists and the head tilts and then more or less locks in place, you are suffering from a condition called torticollis. The problem can be a temporary symptom or a chronic illness. In either case, it presents with pain and discomfort, negatively affecting our daily lives and often carrying an added psychological burden.

Adults who suffer from recurring spasmodic torticollis say that they must endure strange looks and are often treated as if they have less intelligence or are even mentally retarded.

There is no psychological component to a case of torticollis, nor is the condition limited to adults. Children who don't have enough room in the womb or who are delivered breech often develop torticollis within a few days of birth.

Foreword

Their neck muscles have become torn, and when the fibrous tissue starts to heal, it contracts, twisting and turning their heads. Pediatric torticollis is very easy to correct because it responds well to physical therapy and rarely if ever needs surgery.

Adult torticollis is more complex, and can be idiopathic, meaning the cause — and often the resolution — are never given a clear medical explanation.

(Torticollis is not even species specific, but is also common in pet rabbits and guinea pigs where it can be caused by everything from ear mites to toxic exposure.)

All of this points to the intricate design of the human neck and cervical spine. Working together, these structures support the weight of the cranium and allow us to freely move our heads, maximizing our field of vision for accomplishing a multitude of small and large movements every day.

This text is intended to explain the various causes of torticollis in children and adults, and to outline how the problem is most often treated. The prognosis for babies and infants is excellent, but for adults somewhat less certain.

There are people who develop torticollis in mid-life and must deal with it on a semi-permanent basis, an especially common occurrence in those with a family history of the disorder.

Foreword

I am not a medical doctor, and nothing in this text is intended to be taken as medical advice. If you or a loved one has or believe you are developing torticollis, you need to see your doctor immediately. The sooner the problem is detected, the more aggressively it can be treated.

My motivation in writing this book is simple. Torticollis runs in my mother's family. It skipped her generation. She did not have it, but my grandmother did. I barely remember my grandmother, but in almost all of the photographs I have seen of her, she is looking to the side or tilting her head as if asking a question.

This was not an affectation or an intentionally adopted pose. She could not straighten her neck, and as she aged, the condition grew worse. Since torticollis in adults typically presents before the age of 50, I became interested in learning more about it.

So far, I have no signs of developing the condition, but every time I have a twinge in my neck, I wonder if it is a hint of things to come. I hope that the results of my personal research are useful to you.

Foreword

Acknowledgements

I would like to express my gratitude towards my family, friends, and colleagues for their kind co-operation and encouragement which helped me in completion of this book.

My thanks and appreciations go to my colleagues and people who have willingly helped me out with their abilities.

Acknowledgements

Table of Contents

Table of Contents

Table of Contents

Table of Contents

Part 1 – Introduction to Torticollis

The word "torticollis" comes from the Latin "tortus" for twisted and "collum" for neck. In a nutshell, that explains this condition, which you may also see referred to as wry neck or loxia. Breaking down the structure of the word, however, is the only simplistic thing about an ailment that can have many roots.

Presentation of Torticollis

Torticollis presents as abnormal positioning of the head or neck that may also be accompanied by asymmetry of the cranium and facial features. The abnormality may be fixed or dynamic, and present as a combination of tilt, rotation, and flexion. The most typical variant is for the neck to twist to one side causing a tilting of the head. There are both pediatric and adult forms of torticollis.

Pediatric and Adult Torticollis

When torticollis appears in infants, it can be congenital (present at birth) or acquired. The major causes are believed to be intrauterine malposition, breech birth, or cervical malformation.

In adults, the distortion may develop slowly over time or appear acutely after a trauma or as adverse pharmaceutical reaction.

If twisting of the neck appears in people with a family history of the disorder, the condition is called spasmodic torticollis. It appears most often between the ages of 31 and 50 and can become permanent if not treated.

Simply bending or twisting the neck beyond the normal range of motion can lead to acute or episodic torticollis. The person will experience pain and discomfort if they try to turn their head or to hold it straight. There will also be pain and palpable tenderness present in the neck muscles.

Torticollis and SIDS

Although there is no direct causal link between torticollis and Sudden Infant Death Syndrome (SIDS), preventing one can lead to an increased incidence of the other.

Groundbreaking research into the tragic death of babies to SIDS determined that children who sleep on their stomachs at night face a higher risk for SIDS.

Consequently, parents now put babies down on their backs leading to an increased need for children to have "tummy time" during the day. This position forces babies to lift their heads, building the necessary muscle strength to carry the weight of the skull and to engage in a full range of motion.

Although there is no specific way to prevent torticollis per se, ensuring adequate tummy time is certainly key to correct muscular development in a baby's neck.

Causes of Torticollis in Adults

The causes of twisted neck in adults are many and varied. When the condition is spasmodic in nature (also called cervical dystonia) the specific causal agents are neurological and may be related to an imbalance of neurotransmitters affecting the brain's basal ganglia.

The neurotransmitter acetylcholine is thought to play a major role in spasmodic torticollis by increasing the frequency of nerve signals to the region. Ultimately, muscle spasms begin to fire and pull the head to one side (most often to the left.)

Spasmodic torticollis appears gradually, beginning with slight pain at the base of the skull and minor stiffness of the neck. Increasingly, everyday motions cause pulling sensations and pain that becomes severe as the torticollis progresses.

The discomfort is more pronounced on one side, and may radiate into the shoulder, with tingling and numbness moving down the arm and into the hand. The individual may also suffer from head tremors. An episode can last years, sometimes resolving spontaneously only to recur in the future.

Spasmodic torticollis related to neurotransmitter imbalances is, however, only one way in which adults may suffer from twisted neck.

Muscular Fibrosis

An injury to the neck may lead to a case of torticollis due to the formation of scar tissue. Muscular fibrosis refers to the excessive formation of such tissue between the muscle fibers themselves. This results in weakness and fatigue in the muscles with abnormal contractions and shortening.

Muscular fibrosis is also the leading cause of torticollis in infants. If the child does not have sufficient room in the womb the neck may be pushed to one side thus damaging the muscle, which then heals after birth. The damage may also be due to a breech birth.

As the tears in the muscle grow back together, the fibrous scar tissue fills open spaces in the muscle's structure. This growth hampers the muscle's ability to both contract and relax. Therefore, any kind of neck injury, in infants or adults, can lead to an episode of torticollis.

Congenital Spinal Abnormalities

Abnormalities of the spine at birth are not uncommon, and may include scoliosis, kyphosis, torticollis, and vertebral defects.

Scoliosis is an abnormal curving of the spine, which normally forms an S shape when viewed from the side, but is straight when seen head on. In individuals with scoliosis, however, the spine also curves side to side.

Part 1 – Introduction to Torticollis

Kyphosis is an abnormal rounding or curving of the vertebrae that leads to the condition commonly called "hunchback." In less pronounced instances, the affected person merely seems to be slouching.

With torticollis, there is an abnormality of the top seven vertebrae of the neck known as the cervical spine. This is the region of the backbone that not only supports the weight of the head, but is also responsible for the head's wide range of motion from side to side, up and down, and to all rotational points in between.

If one or more of these vertebrae do not function properly, twisting of the neck may result. When spinal abnormalities are involved, torticollis can be more difficult to correct and may require surgery.

The twisting of the neck becomes apparent shortly after birth in most cases, but can present much later in life as the spinal column begins to deteriorate with age.

Toxic Brain Injury - Encephalopathy

A person who has any type of encephalopathy is presenting with impaired brain function. Generally if there is no injury to the brain and no tumor present; the abnormality is due to the presence of a toxin.

For instance, in heavy drinkers encephalopathy may progress to Wernicke-Korsakoff Syndrome, which is a type of early onset dementia.

Part 1 – Introduction to Torticollis

There are, however, many toxins in our environment to which we are exposed not by choice or conscious action, like organic solvents or even chemicals that have leached into the groundwater and thus into our drinking supply.

The classic symptoms of toxic brain injury include dizziness, disorientation, and diminished intellectual skills, but loss of motor control is a definite possibility. This may manifest as an unsteady or shambling gait, trembling in the hands, and an inability to control the movement and positioning of the head.

Traumatic Brain Injury

Traumatic brain injuries are a consequence of external forces causing dysfunction and impairment that is often permanent.

This may come from an actual physical blow to the head or may be the result of being in close proximity to an explosion, a common cause of brain injury to soldiers fighting in Iraq and Afghanistan.

Mild traumatic brain injury or concussion may lead to only temporary functional issues, while more severe brain trauma where bruising and bleeding are present can cause a life time of impairment.

Just as is the case with toxic brain injury, an inability to control the movement and position of the head is a possible outcome.

Scarred or Diseased Cervical Vertebrae

Any injury or illness that affects the cervical vertebrae can alter a person's ability to move their head. These seven vertebrae begin just above the shoulder blades and continue to the base of the skull. Their function is aided by the adjacent muscles and ligaments, with nerve endings interweaving the entire structure.

When problems occur, the issues tend to cascade through the head, neck, and shoulders, with corresponding disruptions in motion and flexibility. A good example of an injury to this region that causes the neck to twist is whiplash in the aftermath of an automobile accident.

Arthritis

Since the cervical vertebrae are one of the areas of the body prone to the development of arthritis, this gradual degeneration of the cushioning discs between the vertebrae can also lead to a twisting of the neck.

This causes not only an abnormal positioning of the head, but also constant pain and stiffness. The good news in regard to this kind of degenerative disc disease is that it actually tends to improve over time.

Tonsillitis

The tonsils are two tissue masses at the rear of the throat that trap germs before they can enter the airway. Additionally, the tonsils produce infection-fighting antibodies. Often, however, the tonsils themselves become infected if they are overwhelmed by bacteria and viruses.

The consequent inflammation and swelling called tonsillitis can cause the nerves at the base of the head to also become inflamed causing short-term torticollis. The twisting of the neck resolves when the infection is treated with antibiotics or the tonsils are removed.

Retropharyngeal Abscess

Although an abscess at the back of the throat is rare, retropharyngeal abscesses are seen in infants and children, but are difficult to diagnose since they occur in an area of deep tissue.

Any time a child displays symptoms including a stiff or twisted neck, difficulty in swallowing, and an overall sense of being unwell, an abscess should be one of the conditions ruled out rather than glossed over.

If treatment is delayed, such a deep-seated infection can be life threatening. Retropharyngeal abscesses are not commonly diagnosed in adults, but they are certainly possible at any stage of life.

Swollen Lymph Nodes

Any swelling or enlargement of the lymph nodes due to the presence of infection or disease can have the same effect on the neck muscles as an infection in the back of the throat.

In some cases, if the swelling is significant, the lymph nodes themselves may impair the movement of the neck. This type of swelling can be caused by seasonal malady like a cold or the flu, or it can be an indication of more serious illnesses including cancer.

Brain Tumors

There are many types of tumors that affect the brain and spinal cord. These abnormal cell masses can be benign or malignant. If a tumor is present, and is growing into a portion of the brain that controls movement or is adjacent to the cervical vertebrae, torticollis can result.

Typically tumors will appear on various imaging scans, which should be performed for an accurate diagnosis of the cause of torticollis. Once detected, management of the twisting of the neck is no longer the primary medical concern, with focus shifting to treating the tumor.

Tuberculosis of the Spine

Tuberculosis of the spine is also called Pott's Disease. It is most often present in the lower thoracic and lumbar vertebrae, but can affect the cervical vertebrae.

The disease causes the cushioning discs between the bony vertebrae to collapse, with subsequent compression of the spine. When this occurs in the cervical vertebrae, it can lead to torticollis.

Ideopathic Torticollis

Some cases of torticollis in adults seem to defy all explanations even when rare factors have been explored. In idiopathic cases, the torticollis often resolves just as it appeared — mysteriously.

So long as life-threatening potential culprits have been ruled out, idiopathic torticollis is more a nuisance than a serious medical condition.

Although the sufferer may be uncomfortable, and may experience limitations in their day-to-day activities, idiopathic torticollis can be managed and is often temporary.

Causes of Pediatric Torticollis

Pediatric torticollis, which typically occurs in the first two months of life, is almost always related to some injury to the muscles of the neck before or during birth.

During the first two months of life, an infant should be gaining more muscle control. The limited range of motion present with torticollis as compared to the increasing mobility of other children of the same age makes the tilting or twisting of the head visibly apparent to caregivers.

The contraction of the muscles is a consequence of the healing process. Scar tissue forms that causes the tissue to contract, twisting the neck and rotating the head.

It is also not unusual for a baby with torticollis to have developmental hip dysplasia, a condition in which the thighbone does not sit securely in the socket of the hip. Hip dysplasia can also be the consequence of a difficult delivery.

In the vast majority of cases, pediatric torticollis responds to physical therapy with no need for surgical intervention.

Muscular Damage at Birth

Whether the damage to the muscle occurs in the womb due to a lack of adequate room, or is the result of a breech birth, the real culprit is scar tissue present in the sternocleidomastoid muscle of the neck.

With first pregnancies, babies typically have less space to move in the uterus, a fact that correlates with a higher incidence of both torticollis and hip dysplasia in first-born children.

The damage to the healing neck muscle in infants with torticollis may be visible to the naked eye as a small lump of tissue at the spot where the injury occurred. Torticollis happens in about 0.3-0.2 percent of births.

Physical therapy stretches the fibers to release the contraction while strengthening the muscles to enable normal function. A TOT (Tubular Orthosis for Torticollis) collar may also be used to encourage the correct position of the head for longer periods of time.

Sternocleidomastoid Tumor

In a situation similar to that which can be created by enlarged lymph nodes, a tumor on the long muscles on either side of the neck, the sternocleidomastoid, can likewise impair movement and distort the position of the head.

Such tumors are the most common masses found on the necks of infants and are actually nothing more than a severe instance of muscle fibrosis. The mass is shaped like a spindle and is not malignant and rarely will a biopsy be required.

Typically the mass will be on the right side of the neck and is more common in male babies. In only 5-10% of cases is surgery necessary to release the tissue. Typically the "tumor," no matter how severe, will respond to physical therapy.

Klippel-Feil Syndrome

Klippel-Feil Syndrome is a rare congenital condition in which the bones of an infant's neck are not properly formed, abnormalities. This is different from other cervical malformations, however, in that the bones of the ear will also be malformed resulting in hearing deficits.

The syndrome is characterized by fusion at birth of any of vertebrae 2-7, leading to a pronounced shortening of the neck with limited movement immediately evident.

Acquired Torticollis in Infants

Acquired torticollis, like spasmodic and acute torticollis in adults, presents in the aftermath of some accompanying trauma or illness. Resolution of the twisted neck typically means addressing the concurrent condition.

Self-Limited Incidents

Self-limiting episodes of torticollis are often caused by exposure to cold drafts or the repeated assumption of unusual postures.

Since infants bodies are still developing, their muscles are prone to experiencing abnormal contractions, especially the sternocleidomastoid and trapezius muscles.

In such cases, a program of parent-administered physical therapy is used to stretch and strengthen the muscles, with the twisted neck typically resolving in 1-4 weeks.

Posterior Fossa Tumors

Posterior fossa tumors are located at the base of the skull and are often responsible for compressing nerves in the region. In instances of acquired torticollis in infants and young children, such tumors should be ruled out as part of a differential diagnosis so that appropriate treatment can be administered without delay. Typically, surgery will be needed to remove the mass.

Throat, Ear, and Adenoid Infections

Infections of the posterior pharynx (including strep throat), ear infections, and inflamed adenoids can all cause secondary inflammation of the nerves at the base of the skull.

Since these nerves supply the neck muscles, a temporary case of torticollis may accompany any such infection. Typically, the twisting of the neck resolves when the infection is treated with antibiotics.

Drug Reactions

Although more rare, drug interactions can also cause transient torticollis. This effect is seen with the use of both antiemetic (nausea) medications and antipsychotics.

The use of antipsychotics in young children is rarely if ever an issue, but drugs for nausea and vomiting are used in this age group. The torticollis side effect can normally be treated with doses of diphenhydramine (Benadryl).

Part 2 – Understanding Torticollis in Depth

Although clear in its physical presentation, torticollis can be a confounding condition in other ways. In infants, it is most common in males. In adults it is most common in women. With babies, the cause is almost always damage to the neck muscles in utero or during a breech birth. With adults, the precise cause is often unknown.

Symptoms of Torticollis

Although the symptoms of torticollis are visibly identical in children and adults, the disease presents in different ways by age and causes.

Symptoms in Children

A visual diagnosis may be all that is required with infants and young children. The child's neck begins to twist and the head turns. The chin will point to one shoulder while the head is tilted toward the other shoulder.

If the condition is left untreated, the face and skull develop at an uneven rate until the twisted neck is permanent and the motion of the head and neck is severely constrained.

Typically, the head tilts to the right and the chin points left. This positioning indicates the affected muscle is on the right side. The child will not be able to move its head well and there may be a lump present on the muscle itself.

Part 2 – Understanding Torticollis in Depth

Symptoms in Adults

Spasmodic torticollis in adults comes on more gradually, and may follow a head or neck injury, an infection, or a course of medication. The condition is most commonly seen in adults between the ages of 25-55 years.

About 5% of the people diagnosed with torticollis report at least one relative who suffered from a twisted neck, with more than 50% indicating a history of head or hand tremors in the extended family.

At first the symptoms are subtle, with stiffness or fatigue present. For instance, you may be driving and have difficulty holding your head straight for long periods of time. It's not uncommon for someone else to notice the tilt of the head first and to ask if you injured your neck.

Over 2-5 years the torticollis will reach its peak, tending not to worsen after that time. The associated pain and discomfort is typically "focal" or located in one place, often the back of the shoulders or the side of the neck.

There are three distinct types of spasmodic torticollis:

- tonic, which turns the head to the side
- clonic, which presents with shaking of the head
- mixed, where both turning and shaking are present

The directionality of the twisting is classified as:

- rotational, with the head turned to one side or the other

- laterocollis, with the head pulled toward the shoulder
- retrocollis, with the head pulled back
- anterocollis, with the head pulled forward

Most cases do not neatly fall into these categories, however, with multiple combinations possible.

Diagnosis of Torticollis

A physical examination will help the doctor to identify affected areas of the neck creating the twisting and turning. Often when the muscles are touched, they will be taught and painful.

If the torticollis is present in an infant, the pediatrician will examine the baby's neck and head. An X-ray will be used to look for cervical abnormalities.

Be prepared to answer questions about the pregnancy and birth. The doctor will also examine the child's hips looking for signs of dysplasia.

Several types of diagnostic tests may be employed with adults since the potential causes of spasmodic torticollis are more wide ranging.

Electromyogram

An electromyogram or EMG quantifies the amount of electrical activity in a muscle at rest and when contracted. The test is administered by a neurologist and takes 30 to 60 minutes.

Measuring the speed and efficiency of electrical signals transmitted by the nerves helps to arrive at an accurate diagnosis for an abnormality like torticollis.

Needle electrodes attached to a machine are used to record the electrical activity. During the test, the needles will be moved to take measurements at different points on the affected muscle.

You may feel a small amount of electrical current passing through the electrodes during the test. There may be some pain and discomfort. The neurologist should discuss this possibility with you and give you the option to take breaks during the test if you need to.

X-Rays

X-rays are a standard diagnostic tool when assessing the cause of abnormal posture. The doctor will use the x-rays to look for partial or complete fusion of the cervical vertebrae, or any fractures or damage to the region.

If the x-rays do not give the doctor adequate information, a CT scan of the neck or even an MRI to rule out neurological problems may be ordered.

Differential Diagnosis Considerations

Sometimes when an individual has been in a serious accident it's difficult to distinguish if the twisting of the neck is caused by acute cervical trauma or if the torticollis is originating from another source.

Part 2 – Understanding Torticollis in Depth

Especially if there are legal considerations relative to a court case for a car crash or an on-the-job accident, it's important that a full differential diagnosis be made. This should include a precise chronological history of the onset of the condition.

Torticollis may be a secondary symptom caused by a primary injury like a concussion or whiplash. Both types of injuries involve rapid acceleration and deceleration which can sprain and damage the neck muscles.

These conditions, however, tend to be accompanied by headaches, an inability to concentrate, dizziness, and blurred vision.

If the abnormal position of the head and neck do not resolve as other symptoms improve, the patient may have what is technically termed "acute post-traumatic torticollis."

In any case of torticollis, however, a whole range of other potential illnesses must be ruled out to make sure that the treatment is appropriate and targeted.

In some cases doctors focus exclusively on the torticollis and miss the real illness, which is likely more serious and indicative of a completely different therapeutic approach.

Other conditions that can cause torticollis include, but are not limited to:

- cerebral palsy
- multiple sclerosis
- myasthenia gravis (Lou Gehrig's Disease)
- Parkinson's Disease
- Tardive dyskinesia*
- Wilson's Disease **

* Tardive dyskinesia is a disorder characterized by involuntary movements of the lower face.

** Wilson's Disease is an inherited disorder that creates on overload of copper in the body that damages the liver and nervous system.

Treatment of Torticollis

Depending on the severity of the torticollis, it may be treated with a combination of medication and physical therapy, or surgery may be necessary to release the muscle tension and restore normal range of motion.

Treatment for Infants

The first course of treatment involves a series of exercises you will perform with your child several times a day to stretch the tightened neck muscle. Either the physician or a physical therapist will instruct you on the safe administration of this therapy.

You will also be instructed in strategies to help your child rotate the chin into correct position. These may include altering how the child is held for feedings, and placement of the crib and favorite toys to require specific movements of the head and neck.

Within a few months, you should be able to see marked improvement of the condition. In the majority of cases, the lump on the muscle goes away, and the child's range of motion reaches normal developmental levels. If this does not occur, surgery may be required or there may be another problem causing the twisting of the neck.

Depending on the age of the child, a Tubular Orthosis for Torticollis (TOT) Collar may also be used. The device is constructed of soft plastic tubing that fits around the neck with firmer plastic insets that sit at the base of the skull.

These pieces are uncomfortable when the child tilts its head, causing a reflexive straightening. Such collars are only used with children 4 months and older exhibiting a head tilt of 5 degrees or more.

Children wearing TOT collars must be supervised at all times and the device must not be used at night or when the child is in a car seat.

Physical Therapy For Adults

Physical therapy is the first line of treatment in all cases of torticollis. The goals are to bring the head back into normal position with an increased range of motion and decreased pain.

The therapist guides the head through a series of movements to stretch and strengthen the affected muscles. This may or may not include a program of at-home exercises.

Heat, ice, and massage may all be used to compliment the exercise.

Medications and Torticollis

Medications do not themselves lessen the effect of torticollis, but may be useful in managing accompanying levels of pain. Almost any painkiller or muscle relaxant can be useful in this regard, and should be prescribed according to the individual patient's tolerance levels and with an eye toward other drugs currently being used.

There are, however, some drugs that can make torticollis worse, including antiemetics like Reglan (Metoclopramide) for nausea and anti-psychotics.

In persistent cases of torticollis, it's important to avoid any drugs that block the production of dopamine. These drugs are typically psychopharmaceutical in nature and are part of the neuroleptic class of medications.

Drugs to avoid when torticollis is present include:

Tidal (Acetohenazine)
Asendi (Amoxapine)
Thorazine (Chlorpromazine)
Haldol (Haloperidol)

Loxitane
Daxolin (Loxapine)
Serentil (Mesoridazine)
Moban (Milondone)
Trilafrom or Triavil (Erphanzine)
Quide (Piperacetazine)
Sparine (Promazine)
Phenergan (Promethazine)
Torecan (Thiethylperazine)
Mellaril (Thioridazine)
Navane (Thiothixene)
Stelazine (Trifluoperazine)
Vesprini (Trifluprozazine)
Temaril (Trimeprazine)

Drugs that may be substituted for items in the list above for those needing these types of medications include:

Cozaril (Clozapine)
Zyprexa (Olanzapine)
Seroquel (Quetiapine)

(These drugs may actually improve the torticollis.)

Botulinum Toxin

One drug that can help to relieve torticollis in adults is the botulinum toxin, which is a powerful poison made from the clostridium botulinum bacterium. It works to weaken or paralyze muscles by interfering with nerve impulses that cause a muscle to contract.

The strain of botulinum used for clinical purposes has been purified and is safe for a variety of treatments from cosmetic treatments for lines and wrinkles to the relief of spasmodic torticollis.

The toxin is injected directly into the neck muscle as an in-office procedure. Generally your physician will first have ordered testing with an electromyograph to determine the exact location for the injection.

The treatment requires about half an hour. After the initial injection, you may be asked to return in 2-4 weeks to evaluate the outcome and to determine if a second injection is required.

Treatment with botulinum toxin for spasmodic and recurrent torticollis usually lasts 3-4 months before another round of injections is required.

Denervation Surgery

In very persistent cases of torticollis where standard treatments have failed, denervation surgery is an option. The surgeon selectively removes motor nerves that are causing the muscles to contract.

The goal is both to normalize posture and to reduce pain. The success rate for the surgery is very high, but not everyone is a candidate, and doctors follow a fairly rigid evaluation:

- Significant relief can no longer be derived from previous treatment strategies.

- The current clinical situation has been stable for at least one year and the torticollis has been present for several years.

- The symptoms are primarily present in the neck (cervical region) rather than in the shoulders and back.

- The torticollis is primarily rotational in nature.

The best success with denervation surgery is to pair the procedure with a post-operative program of physical therapy.

Deep Brain Stimulation

Deep Brain Stimulation is a therapy designed to deliver targeted electrical pulses to areas of the brain that control movement, typically the basal ganglia.

Thin, flexible electrodes are placed through the skull into deep areas of the brain while an external battery is implanted subcutaneously.

Essentially the device acts like a "pacemaker" for the brain. Adjustments are made after the surgery to fine tune the impulses and rate of delivery.

This is a relatively new therapy that is only used in the most severe cases of cervical dystonia that presents not just with torticollis, but also with tremors and severe pain. The surgery is not a fix, but a treatment, and the device requires monitoring and regular reprogramming.

Obviously deep brain stimulation is not appropriate for all forms of torticollis, but for those spasmodic cases that seem to be caused by a disruption in neurotransmitters and that have a clear hereditary component, this approach can offer significant improvement.

Alternative Torticollis Treatments

Not all cases of torticollis are severe, and many are caused by muscle spasm only. This may be in the aftermath of an accident, or as a consequence of poor posture or life habits.

These milder cases can be effectively managed with alternative treatments and home remedies and do not require medical treatment unless the condition worsens to the point that quality of life is negatively affected.

Massage and Chiropractic Care

Regular massage therapy can be extremely effective for releasing muscle of stress not just in the neck, but also in the upper back and shoulders.

If degenerative disc disease and back problems play a role in the presentation of torticollis, chiropractic care can also be useful. Some chiropractic techniques are specifically designed to release muscle contractures like those typically seen in chronic cases of torticollis.

Both massage therapists and chiropractors can also instruct patients in home exercise techniques and postural improvements that can lessen or prevent recurrent episodes of mild torticollis.

Acupuncture

Eastern medicine works on an entirely different perception of illness than that seen in the West. Acupuncture treatments target meridians and channels of energy in the body that, when they are blocked, are believed to be the source of illness and disease.

Like massage therapy, acupuncture has garnered an increasing level of respect from traditional Western doctors over the past few decades for its effectiveness in helping patients manage chronic pain and reduce levels of stress.

The use of acupuncture for torticollis has proven to be more effective in cases where the cause of the twisted neck is directly traceable to sprained or injured muscles. The level of impairment in these cases might be compared to having a "crick" in the neck.

Whether or not the treatment is effective against more serious and chronic incidents of torticollis remains to be seen, but there is certainly nothing to be lost in trying this avenue of approach.

Home Remedies

Some cases of spasmodic and recurring torticollis are more aggravating than debilitating. These less severe occurrences can be aided by a range of home remedies.

Heat application is universally helpful to reduce pain. Standing under a warm shower targets the heat directly on the affected muscle and if the shower head is outfitted with a pulsating attachment, also offers the benefit of a light massage.

Twisted neck can be aggravated by sitting for long periods of time while reading or working at a desk. Try investing in a wearable, battery-operated neck massage device or apply re-usable heat packs.

Try to take breaks while you work, moving your head and shrugging your shoulders repeatedly to loosen up the muscles. Try not to hold a telephone between your neck and shoulder while talking. Use an earpiece instead.

Always use a pillow when traveling or in any situation where you are likely to doze off in a seated position. This not only subjects your neck to an unnatural angle, but to sudden jerks when you come awake.

Buy good quality pillows for sleeping at night, and make sure you are getting an adequate amount of rest. Stress and tension that settles in the muscles of the neck and shoulders makes torticollis worse.

Possible Complications

The most common complications or side effects of torticollis are painful muscle spasms on the side of the neck. Often these strike suddenly and may further lock the head into an unnatural position.

Muscle spasms may also be present in the face, eyelids, jaw, and even the hands. Thankfully, these spasms rarely occur while the person is sleeping.

Adult patients with long-standing cases of torticollis report diminished quality of life commensurate with the severity of their symptoms. Some liken the effects of their torticollis to that in stroke patients or those with multiple sclerosis or Parkinson's disease.

Many of those patients also experience difficulty with depression due to changes in their lifestyle and a degree of social stigma. Patient with spasmodic torticollis say they are treated as if they have a mental defect at times, or are seen as less intelligent and capable.

About 20-50% of long term torticollis patients are forced to give up their current occupation or to alter how they do their jobs.

Prognosis in Torticollis Cases

Torticollis is significantly easier to treat in infants and children with a high rate of recovery in a period of just a few months with little intervention beyond physical therapy.

When surgery is required, the success rate is excellent. One study that looked at a group of patients, age 2-13 years reported an 88% positive outcome from surgical intervention.

Ten to 20% of adults suffering from torticollis recover within a five-year period without treatment and only moderate self-care "remedies."

The rest of the population afflicted with the disorder get gradually worse over five years and then stabilize at a "manageable" level. At this stage the torticollis has become a lifelong condition. It may be stable or subject to flare ups.

In 30-50% of adult cases, symptoms spread to other areas of the body including the shoulders, arms, and hands.

Part 3 – Frequently Asked Questions

While I recommend that you read the preceding two sections to fully understand all the ways in which torticollis can present itself, this section is intended to address some of the most commonly asked questions.

Is there any one cause of torticollis?

Yes and no. All cases of torticollis are, in some way, linked to the sternocleidomastoid muscle in the neck. The muscle contracts which leads to a twisting and tilting of the neck. Why this happens, however, can be traced to many different causes in children and adults.

Pediatric torticollis, which is typically present at birth or in the first couple of months of life, is caused by damage to the neck muscle either in the womb or as a consequence of a difficult delivery. As the muscle heals, scar tissue forms that leads to a contracture or shortening that causes the torticollis.

In adults, spasmodic torticollis may be an inherited condition, the result of a physical injury, the symptom of a deep-seated infection, or even a reaction to a medication. To see a more complete discussion of the possible causes of torticollis, refer to Part I.

What are the symptoms of torticollis?

In infants, parents often have difficulty identifying torticollis, simply assuming that their newborn does not yet have good muscular control. If you know what to look for, however, the "tilt" will be visible within the first week to 10 days after birth.

Adults may suffer from acute torticollis where the neck suddenly "locks" into a twisted or rotated position, or is simply too painful to move out of that position. This is typically the aftermath of a specific injury.

Spasmodic torticollis comes on slowly, starting with pain or tension at the base of the skull that worsens over time. The head may be turned to one side or the other, pulled toward the shoulder, or pulled forward or backward.

What is the connection between torticollis and SIDS?

There is no direct connection, but preventing Sudden Infant Death Syndrome (SIDS) can actually increase instances of torticollis.

Groundbreaking sleep studies linked deaths from SIDS to children sleeping on their tummies at night, so now parents put babies down for the night on their backs.

The child needs a range of neck motions, however, to build sufficient muscles to bear the weight of the head and to gain a full range of movement.

This means that in order to prevent or cure torticollis, the child needs more tummy time when awake to encourage the infant to lift its head for longer periods of time.

How is torticollis treated in babies?

Torticollis in infants is treated primarily with physical therapy and the use of a Tubular Orthosis for Torticollis (TOT) Collar when the child is sitting or walking.

The exercises help to stretch the muscles and release the contracture, while the collar encourages correct positioning of the head. (Note that TOT collars should only be used when the child is awake and being supervised.)

In some instance children who don't respond to physical therapy may need a release surgery, but this is extremely rare.

How long do babies with torticollis require physical therapy?

When the torticollis is detected, the child will need weekly physical therapy and perhaps home exercises administered by the parent until the baby has mastered sitting, crawling, or standing. All these skills encourage the infant to hold its head up and all strengthen the neck muscles.

It's possible the child may require additional therapy on a bi-weekly basis for a few months, but this varies from case to case.

What is a TOT Collar?

TOT stands for Tubular Orthosis for Torticollis Collar. It's a very simple device made of soft tubing that fits around the neck. There are hard plastic pieces located at key spots that are uncomfortable when the child's head leans in that direction.

The device is meant to encourage the baby to hold its head straight and is used in children age 4 months or older that have a 5 degree or greater tilt of the head.

While highly effective, it is imperative that the collar only be used when the child is awake and supervised by an adult. It should never be placed on a child riding in a car seat.

Typically the TOT collar is initially fitted by an experienced physical therapist and adjusted regularly as the child grows. While not a complete solution to correcting torticollis, the collar is an invaluable aid in an overall treatment plan.

How is spasmodic torticollis different from other types?

When torticollis is described as "spasmodic" the cause is typically neurological, appearing in individuals with a family history of the problem. It is thought to be caused by imbalances of neurotransmitters in the brain that affect the basal ganglia.

The condition begins slowly with pain at the base of the skull. The neck begins to stiffen, and over time to rotate and pull. Efforts to hold the head straight are increasingly painful. The condition generally plateaus over a five-year period, but can continue to worsen for life.

When torticollis becomes chronic, it is debilitating and negatively affects quality of life.

Is there any psychological or a psychiatric component to adult torticollis?

No, the idea that torticollis is psychological in nature is extremely outdated. Torticollis may actually be a symptom of much more serious physical conditions including, but not limited to, Parkinson's Disease, Cerebral Palsy, Muscular Dystrophy, and Lou Gehrig's. This can lead to a misdiagnosis and in some instances ineffective treatments, but no doctor should suggest that a case of twisted neck is psychosomatic.

What does cause torticollis in adults?

In truth, there can be many causes, as I discuss fully in Part I. In spasmodic torticollis, the variant that most typically becomes chronic, the cause is believed to be an overabundance of acetylcholine secreted from the basal ganglia causing the neck muscles to spasm.

About 5-10 percent of cases have a hereditary component, with patients reporting a history of the condition in their extended family.

Torticollis can be triggered by an injury or other types of trauma, but it can also present as a symptom of another illness. This is why a complete differential diagnosis is a necessity.

In 15 percent of cases, patients get better on their own with no help from doctors whatsoever.

Are there any statistics for the incidence of torticollis?

There are only limited statistics to track the incidence of the condition in adults. At any given time it is believed that about 125,000 people in America suffer from some degree of torticollis.

If, however, you factor in the impact of the condition on friends and family associated with that person, the impact of cases of chronic torticollis in adults in America probably extends to about half a million people.

Do the symptoms of spasmodic torticollis spread?

An extension of the symptoms of torticollis to other forms of "dystonia" is quite common. Patients often develop involuntary contractions of the eyelids and other facial muscles, and may experience trembling of the head or hands.

Is torticollis life threatening?

Torticollis not life threatening, but it is life altering. In very severe cases where individuals are forced to change how they live and work, depression can be a serious side effect, along with changes in personality and mood.

This always raises the potential for suicide, which is not out of the question with any condition that presents with chronic pain and disability.

What are the treatment options for spasmodic torticollis?

This topic is addressed more fully in Part 2 of this book, but the standard treatments are physical therapy paired with medications for pain management. In severe cases a surgical procedure called denervation may be an option.

Alternative treatment options include massage, chiropractic care, and acupuncture among others. Any treatment is dependent entirely on the severity of the torticollis and the suspected root cause, which may vary.

Part 3 – Frequently Asked Questions

Selected Case Studies and References

The following is a selection of case studies involving torticollis. The condition remains a ripe field of study for medical professions due to its prevalence as a side effect from numerous illnesses as well as a distinct disorder in its own right in children and adults.

Botulinum Toxin in Torticollis Treatment

In this double-blind controlled trial, 19 patients were given injections of botulinum toxin A to improve pain and abnormal head positioning due to torticollis. After the initial trial, an additional 60 patients were brought into the study.

Eight months later, 49 patients reported a 77% reduction in their levels of pain, with improved neck posture in 83%. The most reported side effect across the entire study group was dysphagia, or difficulty swallowing, which was evident in 28% of the patients that received the treatment.

The authors of the study concluded that the botulinum toxin constituted a viable treatment for the majority of patients with torticollis, but the dosage range should be kept at minimum levels to avoid the chance of side effects.

Source: Blackie, J.D. and A.J. Lees, "Botulinum Toxin Treatment in Spasmodic Torticollis," *Journal of Neurology, Neurosurgery, and Psychiatry*," 1990: 53, 640-643.

Outcome of Congenital Torticollis Treatment

The authors of this study set out to identify clinical patterns in the treatment of congenital muscular torticollis during the first year of life in order to determine the effectiveness of given treatments.

A total of 1,086 patients were studied. Of those, 42.7% were diagnosed with sternomastoid tumors, 30.6% with muscular torticollis, and 22.1% with postural torticollis.

The group with sternomastoid tumors showed the earliest presentation of symptoms at age 3 months or less and showed a 19.5% correlation with breech birth and a 56% correlation with difficult labor. Of this group, some 6.8% of patients also were affected with hip dysplasia.

After treatment, 24.5% of patients with less than 10 degrees of rotation showed excellent response to active home positioning and stimulation exercises. In cases with more than 10 degrees of rotation, manual stretching programs showed significant improvement in 91.1% of cases. Only 5.1% of the cases studied required surgical intervention.

Source: Cheng, J.C.Y., S.P. Tang, T.M.K. Chen, M.W.N. Wong, and E.M.C. Wong, "The Clinical Presentation and Outcome of Treatment of Congenital Muscular Torticollis in Infants - A Study of 1,086 Cases," *Journal of Pediatric Surgery*, 35: 1091-1096.

Manual Stretching in Congenital Torticollis

The 821 patients in this study were examined at less than one year of age and were treated with a standardized program of stretching to address cases of congenital muscular torticollis. The follow-up period for the study participants was 4.5 years.

The group was divided into three classifications by diagnosis: palpable sternomastoid tumor (55%), muscular torticollis (34%), and postural torticollis (11%).

Ultimately, 34 of the patients (8%) of the sternomastoid tumor group required surgical treatment, with 8 (3%) in the muscular torticollis group needing similar operations. No surgeries were performed on those patients with postural torticollis.

In 779 of the cases, controlled manual stretching proved to be both safe and effective. The most important determining factors for success were the degree of rotation and the age at presentation.

When surgery was indicated, it was on patients who had undergone six months of manual stretching with no improvement who showed a passive rotation and lateral bending of more than 15% or who had a tumor or tight band of muscular contracture.

Source: Cheng, J.C.Y., M.W.N. Wong, S.P. Tang, T.M.K. Chen, S.L. F. Shum, and E.M.C. Wong, "Clinical Determinants of the Outcome of Manual Stretching in the

Treatment of Congenital Muscular Torticollis in Infants: A Prospective Study of Eight Hundred and Twenty-One Cases," *The Journal of Gone and Joint Surgery*, 2001.

Sternomastoid Tumors and Muscular Torticollis {h2}

In this parallel study, 50 patients presented with sternomastoid tumors and 52 with muscular torticollis. The birth histories revealed a high percentage of breech births with the use of forceps.

In 75% of the cases the sternomastoid tumors were on the right side and there was a higher than expected incident of plagiocephaly or distortion of the facial features. Of the 102 cases, nine had a first or second degree relative with a similar condition.

The study's author determined that the torticollis might resolve completely or manifest as a tumor necessitating surgical removal with the only side effects being minor scarring. The methods described would not resolve facial asymmetry.

Source: MacDonald, Donald. "Sternomastoid Tumour and Muscular Torticollis," *The Journal of Bone and Joint Surgery*, 1969: 3.

Deep Brain Stimulation and Torticollis

The authors studied 12 patients with generalized dystonia and spasmodic torticollis who underwent deep brain stimulation procedures and were followed for 12 years after the surgeries were performed.

Both groups showed significant positive changes at intervals of one and two years. The torticollis patients showed a 59% improvement, with the greatest degree of difference seen in the first six months following the surgery. There was no substantive change after one year.

The authors concluded that although deep brain stimulation is an effective intervention for torticollis, there is no delayed or long-term benefit for the procedure as is typically the case when it is used with other tremulous disorders. Any gains for torticollis patients will be seen during year one only.

Source: Bittar, Richard G., John Yianni, ShouYan Wang, Xuguang Liu, Dipanker Nandi, Carole Joint, Richard Scott, Peter G. Bain, Ralph Gregory, John Stein, and Tipu Z. Aziz, "Deep Brain Stimulation For Generalized Dystonia and Spasmodic Torticollis, " *Journal of Clinical Neuroscience,* 2005:12, 12-16.

Remission in Spasmodic Torticollis

This study followed 26 patients with spasmodic torticollis over a period of 12 years and detected a sustained remission rate of 23%. Each remission lasted, on average 8 years after a case of torticollis that was 3 years in duration.

These findings were more favorable than those believed to be accurate at the time (1984) and were a strong argument against surgical intervention until all other avenues, including long-term successful management were explored.

Source: Jayne, D., A.J. Lees, and G. M. Stern. "Remission in Spasmodic Torticollis," *Journal of Neurology, Neurosurgery, and Psychiatry*, 1984: 47, 1236-1237.

For Further Scholarly Articles See:

Celayir, Ayşenur Cerrah. "Congenital Muscular Torticollis: Early and Intensive Treatment is Critical. a Prospective Study." *Pediatrics International* 42 (2000): 504–07.

Cheng, Jack Chun-Yiu, Constantine Metreweli, Tracy Mui-Kwan Chen, and Sheng-Ping Tang. "Correlation of Ultrasonographic Imaging of Congenital Muscular Torticollis With Clinical Assessment in Infants." *Ultrasound in Medicine & Biology* 26 (2000): 1237–41.

Collins, Abigail and Joseph Jankovic. "Botulinum Toxin Injection for Congenital Muscular Torticollis Presenting in Children and Adults." *Neurology* 67 (2006): 1083–85.

Do, Twee T. "Congenital Muscular Torticollis: Current Concepts and Review of Treatment." *Current Opinion in Pediatrics* 18 (2006): 26–29.

Drigo, Paola, Giovanna Carli, and Anna Maria Laverda. "Benign Paroxysmal Torticollis of Infancy." *Brain and Development* 22 (2000): 169–72.

Giffin, NJ, S Benton, and PJ Goadsby. "Benign Paroxysmal Torticollis of Infancy: Four New Cases and Linkage to Cacna1a Mutation." *Developmental Medicine & Child Neurology* 44 (2002): 490–93.

Gündel, H, A Wolf, V Xidara, R Busch, and AO Ceballos-Baumann. "Social Phobia in Spasmodic Torticollis." *Journal of Neurology, Neurosurgery & Psychiatry* 71 (2001): 499–504.

Hollier, Larry, Jeong Kim, Barry H Grayson, and Joseph G McCarthy. "Congenital Muscular Torticollis and the Associated Craniofacial Changes." *Plastic and Reconstructive Surgery* 105 (2000): 827–35.

Jahanshahi, Marjan. "Factors That Ameliorate or Aggravate Spasmodic Torticollis." *Journal of Neurology, Neurosurgery & Psychiatry* 68 (2000): 227–29.

Joyce, Michelle B and Tristan MB de Chalain. "Treatment of Recalcitrant Idiopathic Muscular Torticollis in Infants With Botulinum Toxin Type a." *Journal of Craniofacial Surgery* 16 (2005): 321–27.

Parkin, Simon, Tipu Aziz, Ralph Gregory, and Peter Bain. "Bilateral Internal Globus Pallidus Stimulation for the Treatment of Spasmodic Torticollis." *Movement Disorders* 16 (2001): 489–93.

Stassen, LFA and CJ Kerawala. "New Surgical Technique for the Correction of Congenital Muscular Torticollis (wry Neck)." *British Journal of Oral and Maxillofacial Surgery* 38 (2000): 142–47.

Stellwagen, Lisa, Eustratia Hubbard, Christina Chambers, and K Lyons Jones. "Torticollis, Facial Asymmetry and Plagiocephaly in Normal Newborns." *Archives of Disease in Childhood* 93 (2008): 827–31.

Tien, Yin-Chun, Jiing-Yuan Su, Gau-Tyan Lin, and Sen-Yuen Lin. "Ultrasonographic Study of the Coexistence of Muscular Torticollis and Dysplasia of the Hip." *Journal of Pediatric Orthopaedics* 21 (2001): 343–47.

Wei, Julie L, Kara M Schwartz, Amy L Weaver, and Laura J Orvidas. "Pseudotumor of Infancy and Congenital Muscular Torticollis: 170 Cases." *The Laryngoscope* 111 (2001): 688–95.

Yu, Chung-Chih, Fen-Hwa Wong, Lun-Jou Lo, and Yu-Ray Chen. "Craniofacial Deformity in Patients With Uncorrected Congenital Muscular Torticollis: an Assessment From Three-dimensional Computed Tomography Imaging." *Plastic and Reconstructive Surgery* 113 (2004): 24–33.

Afterword

Although many cases of torticollis can be improved or resolved, especially in children, the disorder is often chronic and debilitating in adults. It is estimated that about 3 in every 10,000 people in the United States suffers from spasmodic torticollis.

One of the most frustrating aspects of the condition is that it is unique per individual and may waft in and out of acute and sub-acute phases. A spasm may take weeks or months to resolve, and stress and anxiety definitely make management of torticollis more difficult.

In the United States, the National Spasmodic Torticollis Association is a powerful resource for patients, working to increase awareness, offering educational programs, and facilitating a network of support groups. The association's website is located at Torticollis.org.

In the United Kingdom and Europe, patients can turn to the Dystonia Society
at Dystonia.org.uk and the European Dystonia Federation at Dystonia-europe.org for similar resources and outreach programs.

While I am not a medical doctor and this text is not intended to replace medical advice, I hope I have been successful in providing to you an overview of torticollis in children and adults. Often, a critical step forward in becoming educated about any subject is arriving at better questions.

Afterword

I come from a family with a history of torticollis, which increases my chances of one day developing the condition. When I first asked about the odd tilt of my maternal grandmother's neck in old photographs, I was told, "Oh, that's the wry neck. It runs in our family."

I have never been able to conclusively determine how many of my relatives suffered from "the wry neck," or when the trait began in our ancestry, but I was shocked that so pronounced a physical disability would be treated like a benign genetic trait. Dealing with torticollis is not like inheriting blue eyes or a cow lick.

In infants and young children, torticollis responds well to physical therapy because the root of the problem lies in healing neck muscles contracting under the force of invasive scar tissue. In adults, the cause of torticollis is often unknown.

Since there are no definitive answers to the vast majority of adult torticollis cases, I have to leave you with the same mystery with which we began, but I hope you will come away from your reading with more clues about diagnosis and management strategies that will work for you or your loved one.

I asked my mother how her mother dealt with her "wry neck." She laughed and said, "Mama always said she just had a different way of looking at things." I'm not sure if that was a comment on the tilt of her head or a certain pioneering resilience, but regardless, the attitude is commendable for its time.

Afterword

Today, you can get supportive help. If you think you are developing torticollis, don't wait. See your doctor now.

Afterword

Relevant Websites

WE MOVE (Worldwide Education and Awareness for Movement Disorders)
www.wemove.org

Dystonia Medical Research Foundation
www.dystonia-foundation.org

National Spasmodic Torticollis Association
www.torticollis.org

NIH/National Institute of Neurological Disorders and Stroke
www.ninds.nih.gov/

Dystonia Society
www.dystonia.org.uk

European Dystonia Federation
www.dystonia-europe.org

Genetic and Rare Diseases (GARD) Information Center
arediseases.info.nih.gov/GARD/AboutGARD.aspx

Spasmodic Torticollis ST/Dystonia, Inc.
www.spasmodictorticollis.org

American Dystonia Society
www.dystonia.us

Relevant Websites

Glossary

A

abnormal - A condition is said to be abnormal when it falls outside of what is expected or characteristic for a particular patient.

acetylcholine - The neurotransmitter acetylcholine enables communication between nerve cells and muscles.

arthritis - Arthritis is a degenerative inflammatory disease that, in it most common form, causes inflammation, swelling, stiffness, and pain of the joints. There are more than 100 variations of arthritis, which can affect every joint and vertebrae in the body.

B

basal ganglia - Located deep in the brain, the structures that comprise the basal ganglia are believed to play a major role in the voluntary movement of muscles.

Botox - Botox in an injectable treatment developed from a purified version of botulinum toxin A. It is used in small amounts to block nerve impulses in muscles to relax contractions and spasms including those typical in torticollis. It was first approved for use by the U.S. Food and Drug Administration in 1989 as a cosmetic treatment for facial lines and wrinkles. Since that time, it has been found useful in the treatment of migraines, cervical dystonia (a disorder of the neck muscles), and primary hyperhidrosis (excessive sweating).

C

cervical dystonia - Also known as spasmodic torticollis, this is focal disruption of the muscles of the neck and shoulders causing tilting and rotation of the head.

congenital - Any condition, whether inherited or not, that is present at birth is said to be congenital.

contraction - The tightening and concurrent shortening of any muscle.

D

dystonic / dystonia - Repetitive and patterned movements that create abnormal postures and twisted position. Typically occur when muscles in opposition simultaneously contract. The activation may unintentionally "overflow" into adjacent groups of muscles.

F

flexion - A state of bending, as in the flexion of the muscles of the fingers to form a fist.

I

idiopathic - Any disorder or condition for which no direct cause can be detected.

Glossary

infection - An infection is said to occur when the body is invaded by microorganisms like bacteria, viruses, or parasites, which then multiply in a localized area or spread generally throughout the body.

When the body's natural defense systems are triggered to expel the invaders, the resulting symptoms create sickness, for instance fever or the accumulation of pus at the site of a wound.

P

physical therapy - Physical therapy is a form of rehabilitative treatment using exercises and specialized equipment to assist patients in regaining physical abilities or improving physical abnormalities and dysfunctions.

prognosis - A prognosis is a forecast of the probable outcome of a course of recovery from disease or illness.

S

spasm - Automatic, brief jerking movements that can be painful if the muscle clenching is tight.

spine - The column of bony vertebrae surrounding and protecting the spinal cord. The human spine is divided into the following regions: cervical (neck), thoracic (upper and middle back), and lumbar (lower back).

T

torticollis - Torticollis or wry neck is the most common form of focal dystonia. It causes the neck to twist and the head to turn to one side, forward, backward, or some combination therein. Torticollis is common in infants due to crowding in the womb or a difficult delivery, but can occur in adults at any age and for a number of reasons.

Index

Index

infection, 17, 18, 24, 26, 41

inflamed adenoids, 24

intrauterine malposition, 11

Klippel-Feil Syndrome, 22

kyphosis, 14

laterocollis, 27

loxia, 11

Loxitane, 33

lymph nodes, 18, 19, 22

medication, 26, 30, 33, 41

Mellaril, 33

mixed, 26

Moban, 33

motor control, 16

multiple sclerosis, 30, 39

muscle relaxant, 32

muscle spasms, 13, 39

Muscular fibrosis, 14

myasthenia gravis, 30

Navane, 33

neck, 11, 12, 13, 14, 15, 17, 18, 19, 20, 21, 22, 23, 24, 25, 26, 27, 28, 29, 30, 31, 34, 35, 36, 37, 38, 39, 41, 42, 43, 44, 45

neurotransmitters, 13, 36, 44

pain, 12, 13, 17, 26, 28, 31, 32, 34, 36, 37, 38, 42, 44, 47

pain killer, 32

Parkinson's Disease, 30, 45

pediatric, 11, 21

pediatric torticollis, 21

pharmaceutical reaction, 11

Phenergan, 33

physical examination, 27

physical therapy, 21, 22, 23, 30, 35, 40, 43, 47

Posterior fossa tumors, 23

posterior pharynx, 24

Quide, 33

retrocollis, 27

retropharyngeal abscesses, 18

rotation, 11

Index

Index